DETOX YOUR BODY

A Comprehensive Guide to Cleansing
for Optimal Health

Philipp Frühwirth

CONTENTS

INTRODUCTION TO BODY CLEANSING

Body Cleansing or Detoxification has become an essential part of many people's lives. With the current lifestyle that we lead, our bodies are often subject to an excessive amount of harmful toxins, which can lead to various health issues. In response, the practice of body cleansing aims to eliminate toxins, impurities, and unwanted waste materials in the body.

The process of body cleansing involves a range of practices, including dietary changes, the use of supplements, herbal remedies, and physical activity, among others. These practices aim to get rid of harmful substances, rejuvenate the body's natural systems, and restore its balance, resulting in overall better health and wellbeing.

Body cleansing has been used for centuries to cleanse the body of toxins and impurities. Many ancient cultures, such as the Chinese, Indians, and Greeks, used detoxification techniques to keep their bodies healthy, and these practices have lasted through the generations.

The human body is naturally equipped with its system of detoxification. Our liver, kidneys, lymphatic system, and skin work together to identify, neutralize and eliminate toxins that enter the body. However, the modern world we live in, including pollution in the environment, unhealthy food choices, and the use of artificial substances, can overload our natural detoxification system.

The toxicity overload can lead to various health issues such as headaches, skin irritation, digestive issues, fatigue, and mental fog. Additionally, long-term exposure to toxins has been linked to more serious health problems such as cancer, neurological disorders, and cardiovascular disease.

Body cleansing is therefore an essential practice to assist our natural detoxification system in eliminating toxins, promoting healthy organ function, and reducing the risks of developing these health issues.

In this ebook, we will explore various methods of body cleansing, including their benefits and drawbacks. We will also delve into the science behind detoxification, the role of nutrition and hydration during a cleanse, and how to maintain a healthy body after a detox.

With this knowledge, you will be empowered to make informed decisions about your health and improve the functioning of your body. So, let's dive in and learn more about body cleansing.

THE IMPORTANCE OF BODY CLEANSING

The human body is exposed to a multitude of toxins on a daily basis- from pollutants in the air and water to pesticides and chemicals in processed foods. These toxins can build up in the body over time and can cause a range of health issues, such as fatigue, headaches, skin problems, and digestive issues. Body cleansing is an effective way to support the body's natural detoxification process and to rid the body of harmful toxins.

One of the primary benefits of body cleansing is improved digestion. Toxins in the body can impair the function of the digestive system, leading to constipation, bloating, and other digestive issues. Cleansing the body helps to remove these toxins, allowing the digestive system to function properly and efficiently.

Body cleansing can also boost the immune system. The immune system plays a critical role in protecting the body from infections and illnesses. A buildup of toxins can compromise the immune system's ability to function properly, leaving the body vulnerable to diseases. By removing these toxins, body cleansing can bolster the immune system, helping to fend off infections and illnesses.

In addition to its physical benefits, body cleansing can also have a positive impact on mental health. Toxins in the body can cause brain fog, fatigue, and other mental health issues. Cleansing the body can help to clear the mind and improve overall mental clarity, leaving one feeling more energized and focused.

Finally, body cleansing may also help to promote healthy weight management. Toxins in the body can disrupt the body's natural metabolism, leading to weight gain and difficulty losing weight.

Cleansing the body can help to reset the metabolism and promote healthy weight loss.

In conclusion, body cleansing is an essential practice for maintaining optimal health and wellbeing. By removing toxins from the body, body cleansing can improve digestion, boost the immune system, enhance mental clarity, and support healthy weight management. Incorporating regular body cleansing practices into one's lifestyle can lead to significant improvements in both physical and mental health.

DIFFERENT METHODS OF BODY CLEANSING

There are several methods of body cleansing, each with its unique benefits and drawbacks. Here are the most common methods of body cleansing you may consider:

1. Juice Cleansing: Juice cleansing is a popular method of body cleansing that involves drinking only freshly extracted juice from fruits and vegetables for a specific period, usually one to seven days. This method can flush out toxins, promote weight loss, and boost energy levels.

2. Water Fasting: Water fasting involves consuming only water for a set period, usually three to seven days. It's one of the most intense methods of body cleansing but can be highly effective in flushing out toxins from the body.

3. Colon Cleansing: The colon is responsible for removing waste from the body, and a buildup of toxins can cause several health problems. Colon cleansing aims to remove waste and toxins from the colon using enemas, laxatives or other methods.

4. Liver Cleansing: The liver is the body's primary detoxifying organ, and several foods and supplements can support its function. For example, a liver cleanse diet may involve consuming foods such as beets, garlic, and grapefruit that are beneficial for liver health.

5. Sauna and Steam Cleansing: A sauna or steam room can help rid the body of toxins through sweat. This method of body cleansing is beneficial for skin health, relaxation, and reducing stress.

6. Raw Food Cleanse: A raw food cleanse involves consuming only

raw, uncooked foods for a specific period, usually three to seven days. A raw food cleanse is high in fiber, vitamins, and minerals, which can help support the body's natural cleansing processes.

7. Ayurvedic Cleansing: Ayurveda is an ancient system of medicine that emphasizes balance between the physical and mental health of an individual. Ayurvedic cleansing may involve several methods like fasting, herbal supplements, and massage.

It's essential to note that different body cleansing methods work differently, and some are more intense than others. It's crucial to choose a method that suits your lifestyle and health goals, and if you have an underlying health condition, it's essential to seek professional advice before embarking on a body cleanse.

BENEFITS OF BODY CLEANSING

Body cleansing, also known as detoxification, has numerous benefits for the body and mind. Here are some of the most significant benefits of body cleansing:

1. Detoxifies the Body: Body cleansing helps to remove toxins, impurities, and harmful substances from your body. These toxins often accumulate in the liver, kidneys, colon, and other organs, leading to various health problems such as headaches, chronic fatigue, and autoimmune disorders.

2. Improves Digestion: A body cleanse can reset your digestive system and improve your gut health. Eliminating processed foods, sugar, and alcohol can help reduce inflammation in the gut, improve digestion, and decrease bloating and constipation.

3. Boosts Energy Levels: Body cleansing can help to eliminate sluggishness and tiredness, which often arise due to a buildup of toxins in the body. A successful body cleanse can improve the function of organs like the liver and kidneys, thereby improving metabolism, energy levels, and overall vitality.

4. Promotes Weight Loss: Body cleansing can help to kick-start your metabolism and reduce inflammation in the body leading to weight gain. By cutting out processed foods, sugar, and other inflammatory foods while simultaneously nourishing your body with nutrient-dense options, you can support sustainable weight loss.

5. Improves Skin Health: By reducing toxin accumulation in the body, a body cleanse may help to improve skin health. Many people report an improvement in acne, psoriasis, eczema, and other skin conditions after a body cleansing.

6. Strengthens Immune System: Body cleansing may help to strengthen the immune system by reducing inflammation in the body and improving the function of your liver, kidneys and other organs. Additionally, during a body cleanse, you can focus on nutrient-dense foods that are loaded with vitamins and minerals to support your body's immune function.

7. Promotes Mental Clarity: The toxins in our body and our environment can have a significant impact on our mental health. Body cleansing can help to improve mental clarity, focus, and concentration.

In conclusion, body cleansing has numerous benefits for the body and mind. When done properly, body cleansing can help to reset your system and improve your overall health and wellbeing.

UNDERSTANDING TOXINS AND THEIR EFFECT ON THE BODY

Toxins are all around us, from the air we breathe to the foods we eat and the products we use on our bodies. When toxins accumulate in the body over time, they can cause a range of health problems, such as fatigue, headaches, skin irritation, digestive issues, and even chronic diseases like cancer. Understanding toxins and their effect on the body is the first step in taking control of your health and embarking on a body cleansing journey.

Toxins in the Environment

Toxins are present in our environment in various forms, ranging from air pollution to chemicals in our food and water supply. Pesticides, herbicides, and other chemicals used on crops can leach into the soil and water and end up in our food chain. Many personal care products and cleaning agents also contain toxic ingredients that can be absorbed through the skin or inhaled. Air pollution from factories, traffic, and other sources can also contribute to toxic buildup in the body.

Toxins and the Body

The body has a natural detoxification system that works to eliminate toxins through the liver, kidneys, colon, lungs, and skin. However, when the body is overloaded with toxins, this can impair the detoxification process and lead to toxin buildup in the body. Toxins can also be stored in fat cells, leading to weight gain and difficulty losing weight.

Toxins and Inflammation

One of the main ways that toxins impact the body is through

inflammation. Toxins can trigger inflammation in the body, which can lead to chronic inflammation if left unchecked. Chronic inflammation has been linked to a range of health problems, including heart disease, arthritis, and diabetes. Cleansing the body of toxins can help reduce inflammation and improve overall health.

Toxins and Aging

Toxins can also accelerate the aging process, both internally and externally. Toxins can cause cellular damage and oxidative stress, leading to a range of health problems and premature aging of the skin, hair, and nails. Body cleansing can help reduce the toxic load on the body and support overall health and vitality.

In summary, understanding toxins and their effect on the body is crucial for anyone looking to improve their health and vitality. By reducing toxic exposure and supporting the body's natural detoxification process through body cleansing, it is possible to reduce inflammation, slow down the aging process, and improve overall health and well-being.

THE SCIENCE OF DETOXIFICATION

Detoxification is a critical process that supports the body's overall health and well-being. It represents the body's ability to eliminate toxic substances and other wastes that can cause significant harm if not managed efficiently. In this chapter, we will discuss the science behind detoxification and how it works in the human body.

Firstly, it is essential to understand that the body has different strategies for detoxification, including the liver, kidneys, lungs, and skin. The liver is particularly crucial as it is responsible for breaking down toxins and converting them into components that the body can excrete. Additionally, the liver filters toxins from the blood and converts fat-soluble chemicals into water-soluble compounds that can be more easily excreted by the body.

The kidneys also play an essential role in detoxification. They filter the blood, removing waste products and toxins and excrete them through urine. The lungs eliminate toxins by exhaling them as we breathe.

The detoxification process is a complex one that involves several steps. These include the initial breakdown of toxins, which occurs in the liver. Following this, the toxins are converted into less harmful substances through a series of biochemical reactions. These less harmful substances are then either excreted through the kidneys or passed into the blood and eliminated through the lungs.

The liver's detoxification process is divided into two phases, Phase I and Phase II. In Phase I, enzymes in the liver called cytochrome

P450s begin the process of breaking down toxins. This involves adding a hydroxyl group to the toxin to make it more water-soluble. In Phase II, the liver adds another molecule to the toxin to make it easier to excrete. This is known as conjugation, and it involves enzymes such as glutathione-S-transferase, which attaches a molecule called glutathione to the toxin.

Detoxification is not an instant process. It takes time and requires a lot of energy from the body. However, when the body is overloaded with toxins, the detoxification process can become overwhelmed, leading to a buildup of toxins in the body. This can result in symptoms such as headaches, fatigue, skin rashes, and other adverse health effects.

In conclusion, detoxification is a complex process that plays a vital role in maintaining the body's overall health and well-being. Understanding the science behind detoxification can help individuals appreciate the importance of supporting the body's natural cleansing processes through techniques such as a healthy diet, regular exercise, and periodic detoxification protocols.

HOW TO PREPARE FOR A BODY CLEANSE

Body cleansing or detoxification is a powerful tool to help your body eliminate harmful toxins, reset your system, and improve your overall health. However, before embarking on a body cleanse, it's important to prepare yourself physically and mentally to ensure a successful detox. Here are some tips on how to prepare for a body cleanse:

1. Consult with a healthcare professional: Depending on your current health status and any medical conditions you may have, it's important to consult with a healthcare professional before starting a body cleanse. They can advise you on which type of cleanse is best for you and whether there is anything you should avoid.

2. Choose the right time: Pick a time when you'll have a few consecutive days to devote to the cleanse without any major social or work obligations that would interfere with your ability to follow through with the cleanse.

3. Ease into it: Avoid starting the cleanse abruptly. Gradually reduce your intake of processed, packaged foods, and caffeine, and incorporate more fruits and vegetables into your diet. This will help acclimate your body to the changes you'll make during the cleanse.

4. Plan your meals: Create a meal plan for the duration of the cleanse that includes healthy, whole foods. Focus on foods that are easy to digest, such as soups, broths, and smoothies. Avoid heavy, fatty foods that can slow down the detoxification process.

5. Stay hydrated: Drinking plenty of water is important for

supporting the body's natural ability to flush out toxins. Start by drinking at least 8 glasses of water per day and gradually increase to 10-12 glasses per day.

6. Set realistic goals: Don't expect too much too soon. Some people experience significant changes during the cleanse while others do not. Be patient and realistic about the results you can expect.

7. Make time for self-care: During the cleanse, it's important to prioritize self-care and relaxation. Take time to meditate, practice yoga, get a massage, or take a relaxing bath. This will help support your body and mind during the detox process.

By following these tips, you can make the most out of your body cleanse and set yourself up for success. Remember, cleansing is not a one-time event but a lifestyle change. Successfully completing your cleanse will help you feel better and may motivate you to maintain healthier lifestyle choices in the long run.

COMMON MISTAKES TO AVOID DURING A BODY CLEANSE

Body cleansing is a process that many people undertake to rid their bodies of toxins that may have accumulated over time. It can bring various benefits, such as improved energy levels, better digestion, smoother skin, and a strengthened immune system. However, to achieve these outcomes, it's important to undertake a body cleanse properly. In this section, we'll explore the common mistakes that people make during a body cleanse and explain how to avoid them.

1. Starting a cleanse abruptly

Many people make the mistake of starting a cleanse without any preparations. This can shock your system and cause undesirable side effects like headaches, fatigue, or dizziness. Before starting a cleanse, it's essential to prepare your body by gradually reducing your intake of processed foods, caffeine, and alcohol. It's best to start with a pre-cleanse diet that includes plant-based foods, such as fruits, vegetables, and whole grains.

2. Choosing the wrong type of cleanse

There are various types of body cleanses, such as juice fasts, water fasts, smoothie cleanses, soup cleanses, and many more. The type of cleanse that you choose should suit your lifestyle, health status, and personal preference. Some cleanses require a significant amount of effort and discipline, while others are more flexible. It's best to research and consult with a healthcare professional before embarking on a cleanse.

3. Overeating after a cleanse

After completing a cleanse, it's common to feel like indulging in your favorite foods. However, overeating or consuming unhealthy foods can reverse the positive effects of the cleanse and cause you to gain weight. It's essential to reintroduce solid foods gradually and mindfully by consuming easy-to-digest foods like fruits, vegetables, and legumes. Avoid processed foods, animal protein, and sugar for a few days after completing the cleanse.

4. Not drinking enough water

When you cleanse your body, you need to flush out toxins through urination and sweat. Therefore, it's essential to drink enough water, herbal tea, or coconut water during the cleanse. Consuming adequate fluids can also prevent dehydration, which may cause headaches, fatigue, or dry skin.

5. Ignoring your body's signals

During a cleanse, your body may experience various symptoms like headaches, fatigue, mood swings, or cravings. These symptoms are normal and usually indicate that your body is detoxifying. However, if you experience severe symptoms or discomfort, it's essential to listen to your body and consult with a healthcare professional. Don't continue with a cleanse if it causes you physical or emotional harm.

In conclusion, a body cleanse can be a beneficial process for your health and wellbeing when done correctly. Avoid the common mistakes outlined above to maximize the benefits of your cleanse. Remember that cleansing is not a one-time event, but a lifestyle choice that involves making healthy choices every day.

HOW LONG SHOULD A BODY CLEANSE LAST?

Deciding on the duration of a body cleanse depends on several factors. It is crucial to take into account the person's physical condition, medical history, and their ability to handle the intensity of the chosen cleansing method. Here are some guidelines that can help you determine the length of your body cleanse.

1. Start small
If you are new to cleansing, it is advisable to begin with a shorter cleanse to see how your body responds. A two to three-day cleanse will allow you to safely experience the benefits of detoxification without experiencing significant discomfort.

2. Listen to your body
As you embark on a cleanse, you need to pay attention to how your body reacts. You may experience some side effects such as headaches, fatigue, or mild gastrointestinal upset. These symptoms are usually transient, but they may last for the first couple of days. If you experience severe or persistent symptoms, you should stop the cleanse and seek medical advice.

3. Longer cleanses are not always better
You may assume more extended body cleanse results in better health outcomes. However, this is not always the case. The best-lengthened cleanse is one that balances the intended benefits of detoxification with the body's ability to handle the stress of the cleanse.

4. Know Your Goals
Your goals for a cleanse can inform the length of the cleanse. If

your goal is to reset your digestive system, a 7-day juice cleanse may be sufficient. If, on the other hand, you want to achieve a more profound detoxification, a longer cleanse may be necessary.

5. Your Health Profile
Your health profile can significantly influence the length of your cleanse. If you have a pre-existing medical condition, you must consult your doctor before starting a cleanse. Some conditions, such as diabetes or heart disease, require a more cautious approach to cleansing. Moreover, if you are taking medications, make sure that your doctor approves a body cleanse and that your medications do not interfere with the cleanse's effectiveness.

6. Your lifestyle and schedule
Your work and social obligations can influence the duration of the cleanse. For example, if you have an intensive work schedule, you may find it challenging to commit to a longer cleanse. In this case, a shorter cleanse may be a more feasible option.

In summary, the length of a body cleanse should be determined by your health profile, goals, and schedule. It's best to start with a shorter cleanse and progressively build up to longer cleanses if your body copes well. Remember that even a one-day cleanse can offer significant benefits, and the most critical thing is to respect your body's signals and be strategic about the choice of cleansing methods that you embark on.

FOODS TO INCLUDE IN A BODY CLEANSE

When it comes to body cleansing, what you eat is just as important as what you avoid. Incorporating specific foods into your diet during a cleanse can help to support your body's natural detoxification processes, provide essential nutrients, and promote overall health and wellbeing. Here are some of the best foods to include in a body cleanse:

1. Leafy Greens: Spinach, kale, and other leafy greens are rich in chlorophyll, a powerful antioxidant that supports the liver and helps to eliminate toxins from the body.

2. Cruciferous Vegetables: Broccoli, cauliflower, cabbage, and Brussels sprouts contain sulfur-based compounds that boost the liver's detoxification processes and support overall health.

3. Citrus Fruits: Lemons, limes, and grapefruits are packed with vitamin C, which is essential for immune function and supports the liver in breaking down toxins.

4. Berries: Blueberries, raspberries, and other berries are high in antioxidants that protect the body from damaging free radicals and promote overall health.

5. Garlic: Garlic is a natural antibiotic that can help to eliminate harmful bacteria and support the liver in the detoxification process.

6. Turmeric: This powerful spice contains a compound called curcumin, which has anti-inflammatory properties and supports liver function.

7. Ginger: Ginger has anti-inflammatory properties and can help

to soothe digestive issues that may arise during a cleanse.

8. Avocado: Avocado is packed with healthy fats that support the liver in breaking down toxins and eliminate harmful substances from the body.

9. Seeds and Nuts: Flaxseeds, chia seeds, and almonds are rich in fiber, healthy fats, and other nutrients that help support the liver and promote digestive health.

10. Herbal Teas: Drinking herbal teas such as dandelion root, milk thistle, and ginger can help to support the liver's detoxification processes and promote overall health.

Incorporating these foods into your diet during a body cleanse can provide essential nutrients, support your body's natural detoxification processes, and promote overall health and vitality. Along with avoiding processed and high-sugar foods, adding these foods to your cleanse can help you achieve optimal results.

FOODS TO AVOID DURING A BODY CLEANSE

Removing certain foods from your diet during a body cleanse is just as important as adding others. Knowing which foods to avoid will help you achieve the best results and make the cleansing experience less daunting. Here are some of the foods you should avoid during a body cleanse:

1. Processed Foods - These are the biggest culprits in exposing your body to unwanted toxins, mainly because they are high in sugar, artificial sweeteners, and additives. These foods are also full of preservatives that can affect the liver, kidneys, and digestive system. Processed foods also tend to be high in calories and low in nutritional value.

2. Red Meat - While animal proteins are essential, red meat is not recommended during a body cleanse. This is because it is challenging to digest, making it harder for your liver to detoxify your body. Instead, opt for lean protein sources such as fish, chicken, legumes, and nuts.

3. Dairy Products - Dairy products like milk, cheese, and butter can be difficult to digest and can cause bloating and constipation. These foods should be avoided during a body cleanse, as they can also be high in toxins and saturated fat.

4. Caffeine - It's essential to limit or eliminate caffeine during a body cleanse, as it is a stimulant that can increase your heart rate and blood pressure. Caffeine also causes dehydration, leading to headaches and other withdrawal symptoms. Instead, you can switch to herbal teas, which are a great alternative.

5. Alcohol - Alcohol should be avoided during a body cleanse, as it

can interfere with the liver's ability to detoxify the body. This is because the liver prioritizes alcohol metabolism, which can lead to the accumulation of toxins in the body. As a result, the body may not be able to cleanse itself effectively.

6. Sugar - Consuming high levels of sugar during a body cleanse can lead to inflammation, oxidative stress, and a weakened immune system. Sugars found in fruits such as apples, berries, and citrus are still acceptable and highly recommended, but foods with added sugars should be avoided.

In conclusion, avoiding these foods will help you achieve better results during your body cleanse. While the process might be challenging, it's essential to remember the benefits that come with it. You will ultimately feel better, have more energy, and possibly lose weight.

THE ROLE OF EXERCISE IN BODY CLEANSING

Exercise is an essential part of a healthy lifestyle, and when it comes to body cleansing, it becomes even more beneficial. The right type of exercise can help support and enhance the body's natural cleansing and detoxification process. Exercise increases oxygen and blood flow to the organs, which helps them to function better and eliminate toxins more efficiently. Additionally, exercise helps to improve lymphatic drainage, which eliminates waste and toxins from the body.

Here are some ways that exercise can be incorporated into your body cleansing routine:

1. Cardiovascular exercise - Cardiovascular or aerobic exercise increases the body's metabolic rate, helping to burn fat and eliminate toxins. Some examples of cardiovascular exercise are running, cycling, swimming, and jumping rope.

2. Strength training - Strength training builds muscle mass, which helps to improve metabolism and burn fat. It also improves lymphatic flow since muscle contraction acts as a pump, helping to eliminate toxins from the body. Some examples of strength training are weightlifting, bodyweight exercises, and resistance band training.

3. Yoga and stretching - Yoga and stretching movements are beneficial in body cleansing as they help to promote flexibility, balance, and relaxation. Yoga also helps to stimulate the digestive system and encourages deeper breathing, which helps to remove toxins from the body.

4. Outdoor activities - Outdoor activities such as hiking, jogging,

or cycling are beneficial because they expose the body to fresh air, reduce stress levels, and increase the production of the hormone endorphins. Endorphins help to improve mood and boost the immune system, which can help enhance the body's cleansing process.

When engaging in exercise during a body cleanse, there are a few things to keep in mind to avoid overexerting yourself. It is essential to listen to your body's signals and avoid pushing yourself too hard, especially if you are new to exercise. Dehydration can occur during intense exercise, so be sure to drink plenty of water and stay hydrated. Additionally, resting after exercise is essential to allow the body time to recover and repair itself.

In conclusion, exercise plays a crucial role in body cleansing by supporting the body's natural detoxification processes. Incorporating exercise into a body cleansing routine can help to enhance the benefits of the cleanse and promote overall health and wellness.

SUPPLEMENTS TO SUPPORT BODY CLEANSING

Body cleansing is a natural process that helps your body get rid of toxins and harmful chemicals. However, sometimes, the body can use some extra support to flush out some of the more stubborn toxins. This is where supplements come in. Supplements can help support and enhance the body's natural detoxification process. Keep in mind that supplements should not replace a healthy and balanced diet but should be taken as an addition to it. Here are some supplements that can support body cleansing:

1. Milk thistle - Milk thistle is a popular herb that has been used for centuries to support liver health. It contains silymarin, a compound known to have hepatoprotective (liver-protective) effects. Milk thistle can help the liver detoxify toxins, and it also has anti-inflammatory properties.

2. Dandelion root - Dandelion root is another herb known for its liver-protective properties. It helps stimulate bile flow, which aids in digestion and the removal of toxins from the liver. Dandelion root also has diuretic properties, which can help flush out excess fluids and toxins from the body.

3. Probiotics - Probiotics are beneficial bacteria that reside in the gut. They play an important role in the immune system and help with digestion. Probiotics can also help support body cleansing by promoting the elimination of harmful bacteria and toxins from the body. They can be found in fermented foods such as yogurt, kefir, sauerkraut, and kombucha.

4. Vitamin C - Vitamin C is an antioxidant that can help protect cells from oxidative stress. It can also help reduce inflammation

and support the immune system. Vitamin C can be found in fruits such as oranges, kiwis, and strawberries.

5. Chlorophyll - Chlorophyll is a pigment found in plants that is responsible for photosynthesis. It has been shown to have antioxidant, anti-inflammatory, and detoxifying properties. Chlorophyll can be found in green leafy vegetables such as spinach, kale, and parsley.

6. Psyllium Husk - Psyllium husk is a fiber that can enhance the body's ability to eliminate waste by binding to toxins in the gut and promoting bowel movements. It can be taken as a supplement or added to smoothies and other foods.

7. Activated Charcoal - Activated charcoal is a supplement that can bind to toxins and chemicals, preventing them from being absorbed by the body. It is often used to treat poisoning and drug overdoses, but it can also be used as a detox supplement.

In conclusion, supplements can be beneficial in supporting body cleansing by enhancing the body's natural detoxification process. However, it is important to consult a healthcare practitioner before starting any new supplements, especially if you are pregnant or nursing, have a pre-existing medical condition, or are taking medication.

THE BENEFITS OF JUICING
IN BODY CLEANSING

Juicing has become increasingly popular in recent years, particularly as a way to support the body's natural detoxification process. Juicing is the process of extracting the juice from fruits and vegetables, leaving only the pulp behind. This pulp contains fiber, while the juice is packed with nutrients, including vitamins, minerals, and antioxidants. There are many benefits of incorporating juicing into your body cleansing program:

1. Increased Nutrient Absorption: When you juice, you essentially remove the fiber from fruits and vegetables, which can make it easier for your body to absorb the nutrients. This allows your body to get a concentrated dose of vitamins, minerals, and other important nutrients.

2. Improved Digestion: The nutrients in freshly squeezed juices can help to improve digestion, particularly when they are consumed on an empty stomach. Juices can also help to increase the production of digestive enzymes in the body, which can further support digestive health.

3. Enhanced Detoxification: Juicing can help to support the body's natural detoxification process by providing essential nutrients that aid in the elimination of toxins from the body. Additionally, juicing can help to increase urination and bowel movements, which are both important in the elimination of toxins.

4. Increased Energy: Juicing can help to provide the body with a quick burst of energy, particularly when consumed in the morning. This is because juices are rich in essential nutrients that can help to support the body's natural energy production.

5. Improved Skin Health: Juicing can help to improve skin health by providing the body with essential nutrients that support skin health, including antioxidants like beta-carotene, vitamin C, and vitamin E.

When incorporating juicing into your body cleansing program, it's important to use a variety of fruits and vegetables to ensure you are getting a wide range of nutrients. You should also aim to consume freshly squeezed juices as soon as possible after juicing to ensure you are getting the maximum nutritional benefit.

Overall, juicing can be an excellent addition to your body cleansing program, providing a convenient and delicious way to support the body's natural detoxification process while simultaneously providing essential nutrients to support overall health and wellness.

THE IMPORTANCE OF HYDRATION DURING A BODY CLEANSE

Hydration is a critical component of a successful body cleanse. During a cleanse, the body is working hard to eliminate toxins from the bloodstream and organs, and adequate hydration is essential for this process.

Drinking plenty of water is a great way to stay hydrated during a cleanse. Water helps flush out toxins and keeps the body functioning properly. It's recommended to drink at least eight glasses of water per day during a cleanse. However, it's crucial to remember that not all fluids are created equal. Some beverages, like sugary sodas and fruit juices, are high in calories and can defeat the purpose of a cleanse.

Coconut water is another excellent option for staying hydrated during a cleanse. It is packed with electrolytes and minerals, making it a great way to replenish the body's fluids. Other options include herbal teas, vegetable juices, and bone broth.

In addition to drinking plenty of fluids, it's also essential to consume foods with high water content. This includes fruits and vegetables like cucumbers, watermelon, and celery. These foods help keep the body hydrated while also providing essential nutrients that support the body's natural cleansing processes.

Dehydration can have a significant impact on the body during a cleanse. It can lead to headaches, fatigue, and dizziness, which can make it difficult to stick with a cleanse plan. Staying hydrated helps the body eliminate toxins more efficiently, reduces inflammation, and supports overall health and wellbeing.

It's important to note that hydration needs may differ based on individual factors like age, weight, activity level, and climate. It's essential to pay attention to the body's thirst cues and adjust fluid intake accordingly.

In conclusion, staying hydrated during a body cleanse is crucial for overall health and wellbeing. Drinking plenty of water, consuming fluids with high water content, and paying attention to the body's thirst cues can help support the body's natural cleansing processes and make for a successful cleanse.

MINDFULNESS AND BODY CLEANSING

The practice of mindfulness is often associated with meditation and yoga, but it can also be incorporated into body cleansing. Mindful cleansing is not just about what you eat or drink but also about being present in the moment and paying attention to the signals from your body. Mindfulness techniques can help you stay focused and motivated during a cleanse, making it a more rewarding experience.

One of the key principles of mindfulness is being aware of your thoughts and emotions without judgment. This means that you should approach your cleanse with kindness and curiosity, rather than self-criticism. You may experience discomfort or cravings during the cleanse, but recognizing these feelings and accepting them can make the process easier.

Here are some ways to integrate mindfulness into your body cleansing routine:

1. Listen to your body

While on a cleanse, it's important to pay attention to your body's signals. If you're feeling hungry or low on energy, it may be a sign that you need to adjust your cleanse regimen. If you're feeling thirsty, it's a sign that you need to drink more water.

2. Be present in the moment

Staying in the present moment can help you stay motivated and focused during a cleanse. Try to avoid distractions such as social media or TV and instead focus on the positive changes you're making for your health.

3. Practice deep breathing

Taking deep, slow breaths can help calm your mind and relax your body. It can also help you stay grounded during the cleanse, especially if you're feeling overwhelmed.

4. Practice yoga or meditation

Incorporating yoga or meditation into your body cleansing routine can help you stay centered and reduce stress. It can also help you connect with your body and improve your overall well-being.

5. Practice gratitude

Taking a few minutes each day to express gratitude for the opportunity to cleanse and improve your health can help you stay positive and motivated.

Incorporating mindfulness into your body cleansing routine can help you stay focused and motivated, making it a more rewarding experience. By paying attention to your body's signals and staying present in the moment, you can make the most of your cleansing journey.

HOW TO MANAGE
DETOX SYMPTOMS

Detoxification is a natural process by which the body gets rid of toxins and impurities. The process of detoxification can help to improve overall health and vitality, but it can also cause some unpleasant side effects known as detox symptoms. These symptoms may include headaches, fatigue, and digestive problems, among other things. Fortunately, there are several strategies you can employ to manage your detox symptoms.

1. Drink plenty of water: Staying hydrated is essential during a body cleanse, as it helps the body flush out toxins and waste. Drinking at least eight glasses of water a day can help combat many of the most common detox symptoms.

2. Rest as needed: During detox, your body is working hard to eliminate toxins and regenerate cells. It's essential to give your body plenty of rest so that it can devote energy to the detox process. Try to get at least eight hours of sleep a night and take naps as needed.

3. Exercise: Exercise helps to improve circulation and can help to speed up the detox process. However, it's crucial to balance exercise with rest, so don't overdo it. Opt for gentle exercises like yoga, walking, or swimming.

4. Eat light, nutritious meals: Eating light, nutrient-dense meals can reduce the burden on your digestive system, which can help to alleviate detox symptoms like bloating and gas. Focus on foods like vegetables, fruits, nuts, seeds, and lean protein sources.

5. Try herbal remedies: Many herbs have detoxifying properties and can help to support the liver and other organs involved

in detoxification. Herbs like milk thistle, dandelion root, and burdock root can be consumed as teas or in supplement form.

6. Practice stress-reduction techniques: Stress can interfere with the detox process and exacerbate detox symptoms. Try to incorporate stress-reduction techniques like meditation, deep breathing, or mindfulness practices to help you manage stress during your cleanse.

7. Consult with your doctor: If your detox symptoms are severe or persist for an extended period, it may be worthwhile to consult with your doctor to rule out any underlying medical conditions.

In conclusion, detox symptoms are a common occurrence during a body cleanse. By employing these strategies, you can minimize these symptoms and ensure a smooth and enjoyable cleansing experience. Remember, detox is a natural process, and the benefits of achieving a clean and healthy body far outweigh any temporary discomfort.

POST-CLEANSE MAINTENANCE

Completing a body cleanse is a significant accomplishment. After committing to a period of eliminating toxins and restoring balance in the body, it's essential to continue with healthy habits in the post-cleanse period. Failing to maintain a healthy lifestyle can result in a re-accumulation of toxins, which can quickly reverse the gains of the cleansing process. Here are some post-cleanse habits to embrace.

1. Gradually reintroduce foods - After the cleansing period, it's essential to re-introduce foods slowly to avoid overwhelming the digestive system. Avoid processed foods or sugar-rich foods, and instead opt for healthy and balanced meals.

2. Stay hydrated - One of the key benefits of hydration is that it flushes toxins from the body. Drink plenty of water and fluids to remove any remaining toxins.

3. Exercise regularly - Regular physical activity helps to mobilize toxins and flush them out of the body. It also stimulates the lymphatic system and helps to boost immune function.

4. Take supplements - Some supplements, such as probiotics, green tea extract, milk thistle, and CBD oil, can help in maintaining healthy gut function and support liver detoxification.

5. Manage stress - Too much stress can lead to the accumulation of toxins in the body. Remember to take time to relax, meditate, practice yoga, or engage in other stress-relieving activities.

6. Avoid smoking - Cigarette smoking is a leading source of toxins, and it's vital to quit or minimize smoking for the body to maintain its health.

7. Support your liver – As the primary detoxifying organ in the body, the liver plays a crucial role in removing toxins. Support it by minimizing alcohol intake, avoiding fatty foods, and eating cruciferous vegetables such as broccoli, cauliflower, and Brussels sprouts.

8. Practice good hygiene - Practising good hygiene is essential in reducing toxin exposure. Wash your hands regularly, clean surfaces that come in contact with food, and use natural household cleaning products.

Conclusion

Maintaining healthy habits post-cleanse is fundamental in sustaining optimal health. Embracing practices such as regular exercise, a balanced diet, drinking water, and managing stress can help your body function at its best. Remember, body cleansing is not an end in itself, but a stepping stone to better health.

INCORPORATING BODY CLEANSING INTO YOUR LIFESTYLE

Body cleansing is a fantastic way to jump-start your body and enhance overall health. However, to enjoy long-term benefits, incorporating body cleansing into your lifestyle is essential. The good news is that incorporating body cleansing into your lifestyle is easy and can be done without disrupting your current routine.

Below are some tips to incorporate body cleansing into your lifestyle effectively:

1. Make it a habit: To enjoy the long-term benefits of body cleansing, it's essential to make it a habit. Decide on a body cleansing routine and stick to it. You can start with a simple routine like a daily glass of lemon water or opt for an intensive 7-day juice cleanse, depending on your preference.

2. Start slow: If you're new to body cleansing, it's best to start slow. Begin with simple practices, like drinking warm water with a slice of lemon in the morning or adding detoxifying foods like green vegetables, ginger, and garlic to your meals. You can then gradually progress to more intense cleansing practices like a juice cleanse.

3. Incorporate cleansing foods into your diet: A body cleanse doesn't have to be a complicated process. Incorporating cleansing foods like green veggies, lemon, garlic, berries, and seeds into your regular diet can boost your overall health and wellbeing.

4. Be mindful of your diet: For long-term body cleansing benefits, it's important to be mindful of your diet. Focus on whole, natural

foods, and avoid processed foods and refined sugars. Also, stay hydrated by drinking enough water and avoid alcohol, caffeine, and sugary drinks.

5. Focus on self-care: Body cleansing is not just about diet and exercise; it's also about self-care. Incorporate relaxation techniques like meditation, yoga, or massage into your routine to enhance the cleansing process. These techniques not only promote relaxation and stress relief, but they can also boost your immune system and improve overall mental and emotional wellbeing.

6. Stay committed: Incorporating body cleansing into your lifestyle can be challenging, especially if you're busy. However, stay committed to the process, even if it means changing some aspects of your lifestyle. Remember, the more you incorporate body cleansing into your life, the easier it becomes.

In conclusion, incorporating body cleansing into your lifestyle is a great way to enhance overall health and wellbeing. By making it a habit, starting slow, incorporating cleansing foods into your diet, being mindful of your diet, focusing on self-care, and staying committed, you can effectively incorporate body cleansing into your lifestyle without disrupting your routine.

FREQUENTLY ASKED QUESTIONS ABOUT BODY CLEANSING

1. What is body cleansing, and why is it necessary?

A body cleanse, also known as a detox, is a process that helps remove unwanted toxins and impurities from the body. It is essential because modern lifestyles, including poor diets, pollution, and stress, can lead to a buildup of toxins in the body that can be harmful to our health.

2. What are the symptoms of toxic overload?

Symptoms of toxic overload can vary greatly and include headaches, fatigue, skin problems, digestive issues, and recurring infections. If you are experiencing persistent symptoms, it might indicate that it is time for a body cleanse.

3. What are the different types of body cleansing methods?

There are various body cleansing methods available, such as juice fasting, water fasting, colon cleansing, and infrared sauna therapy. The type of cleanse that you choose depends on your specific health goals and requirements.

4. How long should a body cleanse last?

The duration of your body cleanse will depend on the type of cleanse and your individual health needs. Most cleanses last for a few days to two weeks, but some can last for longer periods.

5. Which foods should I incorporate into my body cleanse?

Fresh fruits and vegetables, nuts and seeds, and whole grains are essential foods to include in a body cleanse. It would help if you also avoided processed foods, alcohol, caffeine, and sugar.

6. Are supplements beneficial during a body cleanse?

Supplements such as milk thistle, probiotics, and magnesium can support your body during a cleanse. However, it is essential to speak with your healthcare practitioner before taking any supplements.

7. How can I manage detox symptoms during a cleanse?

It is common to experience detox symptoms during a cleanse, such as headaches, fatigue, and irritability. However, you can minimize these symptoms by staying hydrated, getting enough rest, and practicing relaxation techniques.

8. What should I do after a body cleanse?

After a body cleanse, it is vital to continue with a healthy lifestyle, including regular exercise and a balanced diet. It is also advisable to speak with a nutritionist or physician to develop an ongoing health maintenance plan.

9. Is it safe to do a body cleanse while pregnant or breastfeeding?

It is not recommended to do a body cleanse while pregnant or breastfeeding. Pregnant and breastfeeding women require additional calories and nutrients to support their health and the health of their baby.

10. Can I do a body cleanse if I have a medical condition?

If you have a medical condition, it is essential to speak with your healthcare provider before doing a body cleanse. They can advise you on whether a cleanse is suitable for you and how to proceed safely.